MEGAN DEHOD

PCOS & Parenthood: Your Guide to Fertility Success

A focus on holistic and integrative methods, including diet, exercise, stress management, and natural remedies, tailored to boost fertility in women with PCOS.

This book was professionally typeset on Reedsy.
Find out more at reedsy.com

For Rudie <3

Contents

1

Introduction

Hello and welcome! It's time to move from hormonal chaos to baby bliss! This book will provide you with a greater understanding of your body, how to optimize ovulation, and overcome the challenges of PCOS to achieve pregnancy.

I hope this becomes a mini-guide for women with PCOS navigating the journey to conception, with advice on lifestyle changes, dietary changes and emotional support. When you read these chapters, be discerning and know that you don't need to change everything all of once! I trust you'll be able to recognize what will be the "first dominos" for you— a.k.a the things you should tackle first that will make the biggest difference and trickle down effect in your life.

Follow your intuition and keep your head and hope high!

2

PCOS, Fertility & A Bit About Me

I'm assuming that if you're reading this, you've received a PCOS diagnosis, and so you already know what Polycystic Ovary Syndrome is. That said, do you know the impact PCOS has on fertility?

Ways PCOS Affects Fertility

1. **Irregular Ovulation:** The hormonal imbalances that can happen with PCOS sometimes prevent the proper development and release of eggs.

2. **Egg Quality:** Even when ovulation occurs, hormonal imbalances may affect the quality of the eggs, reducing the likelihood of successful implantation.

3. **Hormonal Imbalance:** Elevated androgens and insulin resistance interfere with the delicate hormonal coordination needed for a healthy reproductive cycle.

4. **Endometrial Issues:** Irregular periods may cause the uterine lining (endometrium) to become overly thick, potentially leading to

2

complications during implantation.

I'm sure reading that doesn't make you feel great. This is what my doctor outlined to me long before I was even considering starting to try for a family.

I'm here to tell you that no matter what your doctor (or anyone else) says, there is HOPE!

There are plenty of success stories of women who overcame PCOS-related fertility challenges to build their families. I am one of them! My doctor told me in my 20s that I MUST start trying to conceive before 35 because I was going to "really struggle" to get pregnant.

I had my beautiful baby boy when I was 33 and, while it did take us 6 months to conceive, that was far less time than my fear mongering doctor suspected it would be.

I'm here to empower women with PCOS to take control of their fertility journey using holistic and integrative approaches. My intention for this book is to keep it short and sweet. I'm here to share everything you need, and nothing that you don't, so that you can begin implementing right away.

No fluff. Here are the things you should do and try before you go the route of IUI or IVF. Let's dive in.

Actually wait...

I'll give you a bit of my story here so you know whether or not you'd like to take my advice.

I received my PCOS diagnosis in 2013. I lived in Europe for a year and didn't get my period the entire time I was there. It was shocking and the first thing I did upon my return to Canada was book a doctor's appointment to find out WHAT was going on. I received my PCOS diagnosis and was told to go on the pill.... And that was basically it, believe it or not.

So, I dove into the research, tried different things in my life and have compiled what I believe to be the most helpful tools.

I'm a registered nutritionist and have applied everything to my own life that I'll be sharing in this book. I've had clients follow similar protocols and lifestyle changes and successfully conceive. I'm not claiming to be THE expert on this, but if this book helps even one person build their family, then writing this will have been so SO worth it.

Before we dive into the changes you can begin to make in your life, I also want to address the emotional toll that beginning a fertility journey has on a person. Every month that my period came while we were trying to conceive, I cried. Every month during the "two week waiting period" when you might be pregnant, I held my breath.

Addressing the frustration and emotional impact of fertility struggles is a very real piece of this puzzle and being able to manage the stress of this journey is essential. This was one of my biggest and "first dominos" in my journey.

Anyway, now that you know how PCOS affects fertility and a bit about me, let's get into the changes you can begin to make in your life.

3

Nourishment & Eating For Fertility

PROTEIN

The most important, and usually under consumed, macronutrient for PCOS is PROTEIN in my humble opinion.

Protein is essential for managing insulin resistance because it stabilizes blood sugar, enhances satiety and supports muscle mass. Combining high-quality protein sources with a diet rich in fiber and healthy fats can significantly reduce the impact of insulin resistance on our hormones.

The biggest thing to highlight here is that the more muscle mass you have, the more you can "get away with" in your diet, essentially. Dietary protein supports muscle growth and maintenance, which enhances the body's ability to use glucose effectively. The bigger your muscles, the more glucose you can store.

How Protein Helps with Insulin Resistance

1. **Slows Down Sugar Absorption:** Protein helps slow the digestion of carbohydrates and the release of glucose into the bloodstream.
2. **Appetite Control:** Protein-rich foods help you feel fuller longer, reducing overeating and stable blood sugar levels help minimize cravings for sugary or high-carb foods.
3. **Promotes Muscle Mass:** Muscle tissue is more insulin-sensitive than fat tissue.
4. **Improves Hormonal Balance:** Protein helps regulate hormones like insulin, glucagon, and incretins (gut hormones involved in glucose metabolism).
5. **Reduces Inflammation:** Chronic low-grade inflammation is linked to insulin resistance. Protein sources, especially those rich in omega-3 fatty acids (e.g., fatty fish), can help reduce inflammation.

How Much Protein Do You Need?

The general recommendation for daily protein intake is **0.8–1.2 grams of protein per kilogram of body weight** for most adults. However, individuals managing insulin resistance, like us, tend to benefit from higher amounts. More like **0.8–1.2 grams of protein per pound of body weight instead.**

HOW To Implement

We want to aim for 30 grams of protein EVERY TIME WE EAT. That should be around the size of your palm if you're having a piece of chicken, steak, salmon, etc.

1. **Protein Every Time You Eat:** Pair protein with fiber and healthy fats to stabilize blood sugar. Example: Chicken or beef with rice and kimchi. (a staple meal in our house)

2. **Start Your Day with Protein:** I'm a big fan of savory breakfasts over sweet to start the day with blood sugar balance. I also think there's nothing strange about having dinner food for breakfast, which is what I often do... last night's dinner = breakfast leftovers. Quick, easy, and more balanced than the majority of breakfast plates. Also quick FYI that two eggs is not enough protein for breakfast. One egg = 6 grams of protein.

3. **Snack Smart:** Treat your snacks like mini-meals. None of this "grabbing a granola bar while heading out the door" type of thing. A snack could be 2 hard boiled eggs and some berries, for example. (Seems more like a breakfast than a snack, and that's the point)

4. **Plan Post-Workout Meals:** Include protein after exercise to support muscle repair and optimize glucose usage. Protein powders are OK if you have one that you like that doesn't give you any digestive upset.

FERMENTED FOODS

Research suggests that individuals with PCOS often have a **less diverse gut microbiome**. The gut microbiome plays a critical role in regulating metabolic and hormonal processes, and an imbalance in gut bacteria (dysbiosis) can exacerbate PCOS symptoms.

How PCOS Impacts the Microbiome

Insulin Resistance and Gut Health

- Insulin resistance can alter the gut microbiome by encouraging the growth of certain bacteria linked to inflammation and metabolic dysfunction.
- High levels of insulin can also affect bile acid metabolism, which influences the composition of gut bacteria.

Androgen Levels and Microbial Diversity

- Elevated androgens (testosterone) in PCOS can directly impact gut microbiota composition, reducing diversity and promoting the growth of pro-inflammatory species.

Inflammation and Dysbiosis

- Women with PCOS often have higher levels of systemic inflammation, which may disrupt the gut lining (leaky gut syndrome) and further alter microbial diversity.

Diet and Lifestyle

- Diets high in refined carbohydrates and low in fiber can feed pathogenic bacteria and reduce the population of beneficial species.

Key Microbiome Changes in PCOS

Reduced Beneficial Bacteria:

- Lower levels of species like *Lactobacillus* and *Bifidobacterium*, which are important for gut health and inflammation control.

Increased Pathogenic Bacteria:

- Overgrowth of species like *Escherichia coli* and other pro-inflammatory bacteria.

Altered Short-Chain Fatty Acids (SCFAs):

- Beneficial compounds like butyrate, which support gut health and insulin sensitivity, may be reduced.

Why Microbial Diversity Matters in PCOS

Hormone Regulation:

- Gut bacteria influence estrogen metabolism through the **estrobolome**, a collection of bacteria that regulate circulating estrogen levels. Dysbiosis can disrupt this balance, affecting ovulation and fertility.

Insulin Sensitivity:

- A diverse microbiome helps regulate glucose metabolism and insulin response. A less diverse microbiome can exacerbate insulin resistance, a key driver of PCOS symptoms.

Inflammation Control:

- A healthy microbiome produces anti-inflammatory compounds like SCFAs, which protect against chronic inflammation seen in PCOS.

PROBIOTICS VS PREBIOTICS

Probiotics and Fermented Foods:

- Include fermented foods like yogurt, kefir, sauerkraut, and kimchi or take a multi-strain probiotic to replenish beneficial bacteria.
- Strains like *Lactobacillus* and *Bifidobacterium* are particularly beneficial.

Prebiotics:

- Prebiotic-rich foods (e.g., garlic, onions, bananas, asparagus) feed beneficial gut bacteria and encourage diversity.

While I believe that protein and probiotics are the two biggest pillars when it comes to managing PCOS symptoms, you also need adequate fat and fibre. I've included a grocery list at the end of this book so you can see how I shop.

I don't tend to recommend a vegan or vegetarian diet simply because most of the protein sources are also very high in carbohydrates, making it more difficult to hit protein targets.

4

Movement & Muscle Building

Exercise directly influences key hormones involved in metabolism, stress, and reproduction, creating a more balanced internal environment.

Exercise increases insulin sensitivity, allowing cells to use glucose more effectively and reducing insulin levels in the blood. Lower insulin levels can decrease the overproduction of androgens (male hormones) in women with PCOS. I'm a HUGE fan of Dr. Gabrielle Lyon and her muscle-centric medicine approach.

This is straight from her website: "As the largest organ in your body, your muscular system is your metabolic currency, your reservoir for amino acids, and it plays a vital role in fighting inflammation throughout your body. Muscle is also the largest site for glucose metabolism, which is critical to reversing insulin resistance and preventing or even treating chronic illnesses such as diabetes or cognitive decline." and I'll add on at the end here ..."**AND PCOS**", because, while the exact cause of PCOS is not fully understood, genetics, insulin resistance, and inflammation are believed to play significant roles.

A quick side note on genetics: I see a lot of people get a diagnosis like this and throw up their hands, giving up because "it's genetics". If you've never heard the term epigenetics before, this should help shift your mindset.

"Epigenetics refers to how your behaviors and environment can cause changes that affect the way your genes work. Unlike genetic changes (mutations), epigenetic changes are reversible and do not change the sequence of DNA bases, but they can change how your body reads a DNA sequence." This concept feels very freeing to me and others I've worked with that have a PCOS diagnosis. This is not out of our control! We can affect our genetic expression by HOW we live and the choices we make.

I believe (and have experienced) that building more muscle has the biggest impact on being able to manage my blood sugar, shift body composition and increase our odds of getting pregnant. **My suggestion for the #1 thing to do in the exercise category is to incorporate or increase resistance training.** ALL forms of exercise are valuable and important on this journey. But if I were to choose our "first domino", this would be it.

I also cannot overstate the importance of postprandial (post-meal) walks. A Japanese study took three groups of men and had them do one of three actions immediately following a meal: sitting, standing, or walking. By the end of the study, they found that low-volume, easy walking for 30 minutes after a meal kept serum fat concentrations 18% lower than sitting or standing after a meal. A.K.A – **Take a leisurely stroll after dinner to balance your blood sugar.**

5

Smart Supplementation

Ok I obviously need this disclaimer at the beginning of this chapter: **Always consult a healthcare provider before starting any new supplement regimen.**

THIS IS NOT MEDICAL ADVICE. I don't know your unique situation. This is what has worked for me and my clients – but I was working with them in close proximity and understood the multiple factors involved.

Now, onto supplementation! I don't believe you need to add hundreds of dollars of monthly supplements to your routine in order to get pregnant with PCOS. These are my top 5, in no particular order.

MYO-INOSITOL

Myo-inositol can improve **insulin sensitivity**, which can restore ovulation. It can also reduce androgen levels, supporting regular menstrual cycles.

Myo-inositol has been shown to increase fertility in women with PCOS, especially when in conjunction with folic acid. When it comes to fertility, a supplement that consists of 2000 mg of myo-inositol plus 200 µg of folic acid taken twice daily for at least 3 months has shown some pretty impressive results. This supplement has been shown to reduce AMH levels and the size of polycystic ovaries better than birth control (Ozay et al.) AND increase egg quality and reduce the risk of ovarian hyperstimulation syndrome in women undergoing ovulation induction (Papaleo et al.).

N-Acetylcysteine (NAC)

NAC improves **insulin sensitivity** and reduces oxidative stress and may work synergistically with inositol, which is why it made this list.

A large study also showed that women taking N-Acetyl-Cysteine (NAC) with PCOS were 3.5 times more likely to become pregnant. What's more, the NAC group also had a greater likelihood of having a live birth and a reduced risk of preterm delivery.

Women with PCOS often have higher levels of inflammation and oxidative stress. Studies show that women with PCOS have almost 50 percent lower glutathione levels compared to controls. Good news: NAC promotes antioxidant activity by increasing the production of glutathione, one of the most important and naturally occurring antioxidants we produce!

VITAMIN D

I also highly suggest vitamin D supplementation, especially during the winter in Canada. Low vitamin D levels are linked to reduced fertility and supplementation can support the regulation of reproductive hormones, including estrogen and progesterone. Consider taking a daily vitamin D3 supplement, especially if your lifestyle or location limits sun exposure. A blood test can measure your vitamin D levels to guide supplementation.

Signs You Might Be Vitamin D Deficient

- Fatigue
- Bone or muscle pain
- Mood changes (e.g., depression or irritability)
- Frequent infections
- PCOS-related symptoms that aren't improving despite other interventions

I don't typically like to give dose recommendations without testing. Speak with your direct practitioner before beginning or increasing your dose.

The general recommendation for adults is 600–800 IU daily. Women with PCOS may benefit from higher doses (e.g., 1,000–4,000 IU) if they are deficient.

NFH PRENATAL

I think The NFH Prenatal SAP is superior to a lot of prenatal vitamin supplements on the market right now. I've been taking this preconception and also into my "4th trimester" and continue to take this as my multivitamin almost 2 years later as I'm still breastfeeding.

The nutrient quality, bioavailability, third-party testing and evidence-based dosages are second to none and they address gaps found in many standard prenatal vitamins. *(I am in no way sponsored by NFH, just a true fan)*

Key Features of NFH Prenatal SAP

Bioavailable Nutrients: NFH uses forms of vitamins and minerals that are highly bioavailable, meaning they are more easily absorbed and utilized by the body.

For example:

- Folate: Contains L-5-MTHF (methylated folate) instead of synthetic folic acid, which is essential for women with MTHFR gene mutations. Methylated folate supports neural tube development and reduces the risk of birth defects.
- Iron: Includes ferrous bisglycinate, a gentle form of iron that is better absorbed and less likely to cause gastrointestinal issues like constipation.

Optimal Doses: Provides nutrients in evidence-based dosages to meet the increased demands of pregnancy and ensure fetal development without risking deficiencies.

Choline Inclusion: Contains choline, a critical nutrient for fetal brain development, placental health, and reducing the risk of neural tube defects. Many prenatal vitamins lack sufficient choline, despite its importance.

Chelated Minerals: Minerals like magnesium, calcium, and zinc are in chelated forms, which are better tolerated and more effectively absorbed than non-chelated versions.

Vitamin D3 (Cholecalciferol): Includes vitamin D3, the most effective form, to support bone development, immune function, and healthy pregnancy outcomes.

Omega-3 Fatty Acids

Omega-3 Fatty Acids reduce inflammation and androgen levels and can improve egg quality and support a healthy uterine lining.

I also recommend the NFH brand here. Their high-quality supplement includes DHA and EPA to support fetal brain and eye development as well once pregnant. That said, if you're eating fatty fish in your diet, you can cover your bases that way as well.

BONUS #6: Magnesium Bis-Glycinate

If you're eating fatty fish, then my recommendation here instead would be a **Magnesium Bis-Glycinate** because it improves insulin sensitivity and reduces stress. Insulin resistance increases magnesium loss through urine.

A significant portion of the population is deficient in magnesium, especially in Western countries.

Why Magnesium Deficiency is Prevalent

Declining Soil Quality:

- Industrial farming practices have depleted magnesium levels in soil, reducing the magnesium content of fruits, vegetables, and grains.

Excessive Calcium Intake:

- High calcium intake (e.g., through supplements or dairy) without balanced magnesium can interfere with magnesium absorption and utilization.

Stress and Lifestyle Factors:

- Chronic stress depletes magnesium, as it is used in the body's stress response.
- Caffeine, alcohol, and certain medications (e.g., diuretics, proton pump inhibitors) increase magnesium excretion through urine.

The pre-natal, magnesium, vitamin D (throughout the winter months) and omega-3 fatty acids are the supplements from this list that I would recommend continuing into pregnancy for a healthy growing babe. Again, speak to the practitioner you're working with and have testing done if you're unsure about adding any of these into your routine.

6

Stress Management

I've saved the best for last, since myself and the majority of women I've coached have the biggest issue with managing S-T-R-E-S-S and yet, this tends to be the last thing we address or change.

Women with PCOS are particularly vulnerable to the effects of stress on fertility due to pre-existing hormonal imbalances. For example, increased cortisol exacerbates insulin resistance, which can elevate androgen levels and further disrupt ovulation. What's more, stress often worsens weight gain, which can amplify PCOS symptoms: a vicious cycle.

How Stress Affects Hormones

When you experience stress—whether emotional, physical, or psychological—the body activates the **hypothalamic-pituitary-adrenal (HPA) axis**, which leads to increased production of **cortisol**, the primary stress hormone. Chronic activation of the HPA axis disrupts the intricate and frustratingly delicate hormonal network that regulates ovulation and fertility.

Disruption of the Hypothalamic-Pituitary-Ovarian (HPO) Axis:

- The HPO axis controls the release of key reproductive hormones:
- **Gonadotropin-releasing hormone (GnRH):** Stimulates the release of follicle-stimulating hormone (FSH) and luteinizing hormone (LH).
- **FSH:** Promotes ovarian follicle development.
- **LH:** Triggers ovulation.
- Chronic stress suppresses GnRH, leading to irregular or absent ovulation (**anovulation**) and disrupted menstrual cycles.

Elevated Cortisol Levels:

- High cortisol competes with progesterone for its receptors, which can lower progesterone availability, essential for maintaining the luteal phase and supporting early pregnancy.
- Elevated cortisol also suppresses estrogen, further impairing ovulation.

Increased Prolactin Production:

- Stress can elevate prolactin levels, which in excess can inhibit ovulation and lead to irregular menstrual cycles (a condition called hyperprolactinemia).

Impact on Insulin Sensitivity:

- Stress can worsen insulin resistance, further disrupting ovulation and hormone balance.

Thyroid Hormone Disruption:

- Chronic stress can suppress thyroid function, leading to hypothyroidism, which is linked to menstrual irregularities and infertility.
-

I feel like at this point we've all tried some form of mindfulness meditation, deep breathing exercise, and journaling or affirmations practice. Those things are all wonderful, and if you haven't tried some or all of them, please do. That said, I'll share some practices that have been helpful for me in my journey that aren't "the typical."

Personally, I like to focus on somatic practice because they address the physical sensations and embodied experience of stress, rather than focusing solely on the mind. Somatic practices are body-focused techniques that help reduce stress by calming the nervous system and releasing tension stored in the body.

1. Progressive Muscle Relaxation (PMR)

- Focus: Reduces physical tension by systematically tensing and relaxing muscle groups.
- How to Practice:

1. Sit or lie in a quiet space.
2. Starting with your feet, tense the muscles for 5–7 seconds, then release completely.
3. Move upward through your body (legs, abdomen, arms, shoulders, face), repeating the process.
4. Notice the contrast between tension and relaxation.

2. Grounding Techniques

- Focus: Anchors you in the present moment to reduce anxiety.
- Practices:
- **5-4-3-2-1 Method:** Identify 5 things you see, 4 things you feel, 3 things you hear, 2 things you smell, and 1 thing you taste.
- **Barefoot Grounding:** Walk barefoot on grass, sand, or soil to connect physically with the earth and discharge built-up tension.

3. Vagus Nerve Stimulation

- Focus: Activates the parasympathetic nervous system to counteract stress.
- Practices:
- **Humming or Singing:** Vibrations from vocalizing stimulate the vagus nerve.
- **Cold Exposure:** Splash cold water on your face or apply a cold compress to the back of your neck.
- **Gargling:** Stimulates the vagus nerve and promotes relaxation.

4. Tapping (EFT - Emotional Freedom Techniques)

- Focus: Combines gentle tapping on acupressure points with affirmations to reduce stress.
- How to Practice:

1. Tap lightly on specific points (e.g., top of the head, eyebrows, under the eyes, collarbone) while focusing on a stressful thought or emotion.
2. Pair the tapping with calming affirmations, such as, "Even though I feel stressed, I deeply accept myself."

5. Dynamic Shaking (Shaking Therapy)

- Focus: Releases tension and pent-up energy from the body.
- How to Practice:

1. Stand with your feet hip-width apart.
2. Begin shaking your arms, legs, and torso gently, letting the movement flow naturally.
3. Gradually increase the intensity for 2–3 minutes, then slow down and pause to feel the sensations in your body.

All of these practices can shift the nervous system from the **sympathetic (fight-or-flight)** state to the **parasympathetic (rest-and-digest)** state, which is where we want to be FAR more often.

Practices like Yin Yoga or restorative yoga that emphasize slow movements and deep stretches can also be added into your week. Schedule it in. If you're like me, if it's not in the calendar, it won't get done!

Integrating stress-reducing strategies can significantly improve the likelihood of conception and overall reproductive health. The mind-body connection is no joke!

7

Conclusion

As you begin your journey, and perhaps implement some of what is in this book, it's so important to prioritize emotional wellness and try to build a support system around you. It can truly be a roller coaster managing feelings of frustration, hope, and grief each month. Friends, family and connecting with support groups and online communities can help. Be open and honest with your partner throughout.

Reach out to me on social media – I'm always happy to chat. And of course, message me when you've got your little bun in the oven!

If you found this book helpful, I'd be very appreciative if you left a favorable review for it on Amazon. Thank you for reading!

8

References

1. Centers for Disease Control and Prevention (CDC). (n.d.). *Epigenetic impacts on health.* Retrieved from https://www.cdc.gov/genomics-and-health/about/epigenetic-impacts-on-health.html

2. Gabrielle Lyon. (n.d.). *Dr. Gabrielle Lyon's website.* Retrieved from https://drgabriellelyon.com/

3. NFH. (n.d.). *Prenatal SAP - 180 capsules.* Retrieved from https://shopnfh.ca/prenatal-sap-180-capsules

4. Rizal, B., Karmin, C., & Villanueva, C. M. (2021). PCOS and its effects on metabolic disorders. *Journal of Medicine, Surgery & Trauma (JMUST).* Retrieved from https://jmust.org/elib/journal/doi/10.35460/2546-1621.2021-0141/full

5. Rosenfield, R. L., Ehrmann, D. A., & Hoeger, K. M. (2024). Advances in the diagnosis and treatment of PCOS. *The Journal of Clinical Endocrinology & Metabolism, 109*(6), 1630–1642. Retrieved from https://academic.oup.com/jcem/article/109/6/1630/7504796?login=false

6. Yin, J., & Xu, Z. (2024). New insights into the role of inflammation in PCOS. *Frontiers in Endocrinology.* Retrieved from https://www.fr

ontiersin.org/journals/endocrinology/articles/10.3389/fendo.202
4.1456571/full

7. Today's Dietitian. (2017). *New data on polycystic ovary syndrome.*
   Retrieved from https://www.todaysdietitian.com/newarchives/05
   17p12.shtml

8. Unfer, V., Carlomagno, G., Rizzo, P., & Roseff, S. (2012). Myo-
   inositol in the treatment of polycystic ovary syndrome: A review
   of the evidence. *Journal of Endocrinological Investigation, 35*(11),
   1029–1035. Retrieved from https://pubmed.ncbi.nlm.nih.gov/228
   95871/

9

PCOS-Friendly Grocery List

This list is designed to help manage **insulin resistance**, **inflammation**, and **hormonal imbalances**. It focuses on whole, nutrient-dense foods that support blood sugar stability and gut health.

Proteins

- **Animal Protein:** *(grass-fed, wild-caught and pasture-raised whenever possible) *make friends with a local farmer!*
- Chicken
- Turkey
- Salmon
- Sardines
- Beef
- Eggs

Healthy Fats

- **Oils:**
- Extra virgin olive oil
- Avocado oil
- Coconut oil
- **Fats:**
- Avocados
- Nuts (almonds, walnuts, Brazil nuts)
- Seeds (chia seeds, flaxseeds, pumpkin seeds, sunflower seeds)
- Nut butters (unsweetened, natural)

Complex Carbohydrates

Grains:

- Rice
- Oats (steel–cut or rolled)
- Buckwheat

Starchy Vegetables:

- Sweet potatoes
- Butternut squash
- Pumpkin

Non–Starchy Vegetables (Low–Glycemic Index)

Leafy Greens:

- Spinach

- Kale
- Swiss chard
- Arugula

Cruciferous Vegetables:

- Broccoli
- Cauliflower
- Brussels sprouts
- Cabbage

Other Vegetables:

- Zucchini
- Bell peppers
- Mushrooms
- Eggplant
- Asparagus
- Green beans
- Celery
- Cucumber

Low-Glycemic Fruits

- Berries (blueberries, raspberries, strawberries, blackberries)
- Apples
- Pears
- Oranges
- Grapefruit
- Kiwi
- Pomegranate

- Cherries

Dairy (& dairy alternatives)

- Unsweetened coconut milk
- Plain Greek yogurt (low-fat or full-fat, depending on preference)
- Hard cheeses (e.g., Parmesan, aged cheddar, in moderation)

Herbs, Spices, and Flavorings

- Fresh herbs (parsley, cilantro, basil, mint)
- Spices (turmeric, cinnamon, ginger, cumin, paprika)
- Apple cider vinegar
- Lemon and lime
- Garlic
- Hot sauce (Frank's Red Hot, Sriracha)

Beverages

- Herbal teas (spearmint tea for reducing androgens, chamomile for stress relief)
- Water
- Bone broth (for gut health)

Snacks and Pantry Staples

- Dark chocolate (70% cocoa or higher)
- Olives
- Hummus (pair with veggies)
- Rice cakes (topped with avocado or nut butter)
- Seaweed snacks

- Popcorn (air-popped)

I also want to just note that there are no foods you "can't" eat. The amount of fear mongering in the health space is absolutely wild.

Fruit is bad, meat is bad, grains are the devil.

No wonder people are confused and overwhelmed and disconnected on how to eat and nourish themselves.

I spend a lot of time in my practice dispelling nutrition myths and bringing people to a place of ease and balance when it comes to nutrition.

If you are eating whole foods, most of the time, you are doing AMAZING. I find there is way too much focus on the nuance and not enough zoomed out conversations on the bigger picture when it comes to nutrition and health.

You do not need to cut out entire food groups to get pregnant. What I would prioritize is a:

- **Focus on Whole Foods:** Avoid processed and refined foods as much as possible.
- **Choose Low-Glycemic Options:** Stick to foods that help maintain stable blood sugar levels. And ENJOY!

www.ingramcontent.com/pod-product-compliance
Lightning Source LLC
Chambersburg PA
CBHW051719250726
48653CB00008B/3102